90-day Wellness Planner

Dr. Lana Moshkovich's

90-day Wellness Planner / Dr. Lana Moshkovich

This wellness planner belongs to:

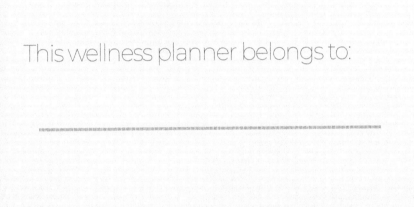

I intend to feel energized and motivated as I follow Dr. Lana's Weight Loss Workbook..

My success and happiness is a result of the dedicated work I put in to reach my goals.

Many weight loss programs require you to follow a specific diet. Some of the programs include supplements and/ or medication. Majority of weight loss programs limit certain nutrients groups, like fat, carbohydrates or protein. Many programs promise fast results and it can cost up to $9k for 6 month.

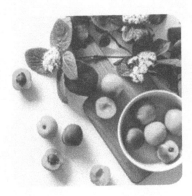

Our Weight Loss Program is for the serious and committed.

If you want to lose and maintain your desired healthy weight then this program is for you.

https://www.nirvananaturopathics.com/contents/ programs/weight-loss-mentorship

Day _____

Weight _____   BMI _____   Size _____

My mood   Drink water

☹ ☹ 😐 🙂 😄   ∀∀∀∀∀∀

What can I do to feel better today
_____
_____
_____
_____

Affirmation
_____
_____
_____
_____

Notes
_____
_____
_____

Exercise

https://youtu.be/gndCthN8SlY

Schedule

5:00 _____
5:30 _____
6:00 _____
6:30 _____
7:00 _____
7:30 _____
8:00 _____
8:30 _____
9:00 _____
9:30 _____
10:00 _____
10:30 _____
11:00 _____
11:30 _____
12:00 _____
12:30 _____
1:00 _____
1:30 _____
2:00 _____
2:30 _____
3:00 _____
3:30 _____
4:00 _____
4:30 _____
5:00 _____
5:30 _____
6:00 _____
6:30 _____
7:00 _____
7:30 _____
8:00 _____
8:30 _____
9:00 _____
9:30 _____
10:00 _____
10:30 _____
11:00 _____
11:30 _____

Morning brainstorm

Big Goals

Extra Goals

Evening reflection

Day

Weight _____   BMI _____   Size _____

My mood   Drink water

☹ ☹ 😐 🙂 😃   ⊔ ⊔ ⊔ ⊔ ⊔ ⊔

What can I do to feel better today

Affirmation

Notes

https://youtu.be/AVRYrrrQeds

Exercise

Schedule

Time	
5:00	
5:30	
6:00	
6:30	
7:00	
7:30	
8:00	
8:30	
9:00	
9:30	
10:00	
10:30	
11:00	
11:30	
12:00	
12:30	
1:00	
1:30	
2:00	
2:30	
3:00	
3:30	
4:00	
4:30	
5:00	
5:30	
6:00	
6:30	
7:00	
7:30	
8:00	
8:30	
9:00	
9:30	
10:00	
10:30	
11:00	
11:30	

Morning brainstorm

Big Goals

Extra Goals

Evening reflection

Day

Weight _____   BMI _____   Size _____

My mood   Drink water

☹ ☹ 😐 🙂 😃   ⊔ ⊔ ⊔ ⊔ ⊔ ⊔ ⊔

What can I do to feel better today

_____
_____
_____
_____

Affirmation

_____
_____
_____
_____

Notes

_____
_____
_____
_____

https://youtu.be/k7iq2Z2D1Zs

Exercise

Schedule

5:00 _____
5:30 _____
6:00 _____
6:30 _____
7:00 _____
7:30 _____
8:00 _____
8:30 _____
9:00 _____
9:30 _____
10:00 _____
10:30 _____
11:00 _____
11:30 _____
12:00 _____
12:30 _____
1:00 _____
1:30 _____
2:00 _____
2:30 _____
3:00 _____
3:30 _____
4:00 _____
4:30 _____
5:00 _____
5:30 _____
6:00 _____
6:30 _____
7:00 _____
7:30 _____
8:00 _____
8:30 _____
9:00 _____
9:30 _____
10:00 _____
10:30 _____
11:00 _____
11:30 _____

Morning brainstorm

Big Goals

Extra Goals

Evening reflection

Day

Weight _____ BMI _____ Size _____

My mood

☹ ☹ 😐 🙂 😃

Drink water

⊔⊔⊔⊔⊔⊔⊔

What can I do to feel better today
_____
_____
_____
_____

Affirmation
_____
_____
_____
_____

Notes
_____
_____
_____
_____

Exercise

Schedule

Time	
5:00	
5:30	
6:00	
6:30	
7:00	
7:30	
8:00	
8:30	
9:00	
9:30	
10:00	
10:30	
11:00	
11:30	
12:00	
12:30	
1:00	
1:30	
2:00	
2:30	
3:00	
3:30	
4:00	
4:30	
5:00	
5:30	
6:00	
6:30	
7:00	
7:30	
8:00	
8:30	
9:00	
9:30	
10:00	
10:30	
11:00	
11:30	

Morning brainstorm

Big Goals

Extra Goals

Evening reflection

Day

Weight _____ BMI _____ Size _____

My mood   Drink water

☹ ☹ 😐 🙂 😀   ᶣ ᶣ ᶣ ᶣ ᶣ ᶣ

What can I do to feel better today
_____
_____
_____
_____

Affirmation
_____
_____
_____
_____

Notes
_____
_____
_____
_____

Exercise

Schedule

5:00	
5:30	
6:00	
6:30	
7:00	
7:30	
8:00	
8:30	
9:00	
9:30	
10:00	
10:30	
11:00	
11:30	
12:00	
12:30	
1:00	
1:30	
2:00	
2:30	
3:00	
3:30	
4:00	
4:30	
5:00	
5:30	
6:00	
6:30	
7:00	
7:30	
8:00	
8:30	
9:00	
9:30	
10:00	
10:30	
11:00	
11:30	

Morning brainstorm

Big Goals

Extra Goals

Evening reflection

Day

Weight _____   BMI _____   Size _____

My mood   Drink water

☹ ☹ 😐 🙂 😀   ⊔ ⊔ ⊔ ⊔ ⊔ ⊔

What can I do to feel better today

Affirmation

Notes

Exercise

Schedule

Time	
5:00	
5:30	
6:00	
6:30	
7:00	
7:30	
8:00	
8:30	
9:00	
9:30	
10:00	
10:30	
11:00	
11:30	
12:00	
12:30	
1:00	
1:30	
2:00	
2:30	
3:00	
3:30	
4:00	
4:30	
5:00	
5:30	
6:00	
6:30	
7:00	
7:30	
8:00	
8:30	
9:00	
9:30	
10:00	
10:30	
11:00	
11:30	

Morning brainstorm

Big Goals

Extra Goals

Evening reflection

Day _____

Weight _____ BMI _____ Size _____

My mood

😞 😟 😐 🙂 😃

Drink water

⊌ ⊌ ⊌ ⊌ ⊌ ⊌

What can I do to feel better today

_____
_____
_____

Affirmation

_____
_____
_____

Notes

_____
_____
_____

Exercise

https://youtu.be/cqwQosiUhTk

Schedule

Time	
5:00	
5:30	
6:00	
6:30	
7:00	
7:30	
8:00	
8:30	
9:00	
9:30	
10:00	
10:30	
11:00	
11:30	
12:00	
12:30	
1:00	
1:30	
2:00	
2:30	
3:00	
3:30	
4:00	
4:30	
5:00	
5:30	
6:00	
6:30	
7:00	
7:30	
8:00	
8:30	
9:00	
9:30	
10:00	
10:30	
11:00	
11:30	

Morning brainstorm

Big Goals

Extra Goals

Evening reflection

Day

Weight _____ BMI _____ Size _____

My mood   Drink water

☹ ☹ 😐 ☺ 😃   ⊔⊔⊔⊔⊔⊔

What can I do to feel better today

Affirmation

Notes

Exercise

Schedule

Time	
5:00	
5:30	
6:00	
6:30	
7:00	
7:30	
8:00	
8:30	
9:00	
9:30	
10:00	
10:30	
11:00	
11:30	
12:00	
12:30	
1:00	
1:30	
2:00	
2:30	
3:00	
3:30	
4:00	
4:30	
5:00	
5:30	
6:00	
6:30	
7:00	
7:30	
8:00	
8:30	
9:00	
9:30	
10:00	
10:30	
11:00	
11:30	

Morning brainstorm

Big Goals

Extra Goals

Evening reflection

Day _____

Weight _____   BMI _____   Size _____

My mood

Drink water

What can I do to feel better today

Affirmation

Notes

Exercise

https://youtu.be/Bet7pI3p4_g

Schedule

5:00
5:30
6:00
6:30
7:00
7:30
8:00
8:30
9:00
9:30
10:00
10:30
11:00
11:30
12:00
12:30
1:00
1:30
2:00
2:30
3:00
3:30
4:00
4:30
5:00
5:30
6:00
6:30
7:00
7:30
8:00
8:30
9:00
9:30
10:00
10:30
11:00
11:30

Morning brainstorm

Big Goals

Extra Goals

Evening reflection

Day _____

Weight _____ BMI _____ Size _____

My mood

☹ ☹ 😐 🙂 😄

Drink water

⊔ ⊔ ⊔ ⊔ ⊔ ⊔

What can I do to feel better today
_____
_____
_____
_____

Affirmation
_____
_____
_____
_____

Notes
_____
_____
_____
_____

Stand
16/12 hours

12:00   6:00   NOON   6:00

Awards

Exercise

Schedule

Time	
5:00	
5:30	
6:00	
6:30	
7:00	
7:30	
8:00	
8:30	
9:00	
9:30	
10:00	
10:30	
11:00	
11:30	
12:00	
12:30	
1:00	
1:30	
2:00	
2:30	
3:00	
3:30	
4:00	
4:30	
5:00	
5:30	
6:00	
6:30	
7:00	
7:30	
8:00	
8:30	
9:00	
9:30	
10:00	
10:30	
11:00	
11:30	

Morning brainstorm

Big Goals

Extra Goals

Evening reflection

Day

Weight _____ BMI _____ Size _____

My mood

☹ ☹ 😐 🙂 😄

Drink water

⛶ ⛶ ⛶ ⛶ ⛶ ⛶

What can I do to feel better today
_____
_____
_____

Affirmation
_____
_____
_____

Notes
_____
_____
_____

Exercise

Schedule

5:00 _____
5:30 _____
6:00 _____
6:30 _____
7:00 _____
7:30 _____
8:00 _____
8:30 _____
9:00 _____
9:30 _____
10:00 _____
10:30 _____
11:00 _____
11:30 _____
12:00 _____
12:30 _____
1:00 _____
1:30 _____
2:00 _____
2:30 _____
3:00 _____
3:30 _____
4:00 _____
4:30 _____
5:00 _____
5:30 _____
6:00 _____
6:30 _____
7:00 _____
7:30 _____
8:00 _____
8:30 _____
9:00 _____
9:30 _____
10:00 _____
10:30 _____
11:00 _____
11:30 _____

Morning brainstorm

Big Goals

Extra Goals

Evening reflection

Day

Weight _____ BMI _____ Size _____

My mood

☹ ☹ 😐 🙂 😃

Drink water

🥤🥤🥤🥤🥤🥤

What can I do to feel better today

Affirmation

Notes

Exercise

Schedule

5:00	
5:30	
6:00	
6:30	
7:00	
7:30	
8:00	
8:30	
9:00	
9:30	
10:00	
10:30	
11:00	
11:30	
12:00	
12:30	
1:00	
1:30	
2:00	
2:30	
3:00	
3:30	
4:00	
4:30	
5:00	
5:30	
6:00	
6:30	
7:00	
7:30	
8:00	
8:30	
9:00	
9:30	
10:00	
10:30	
11:00	
11:30	

Morning brainstorm

Big Goals

Extra Goals

Evening reflection

Day

Weight _____   BMI _____   Size _____

My mood   Drink water

☹ ☹ 😐 🙂 😃   ᗺ ᗺ ᗺ ᗺ ᗺ ᗺ

What can I do to feel better today

Affirmation

Notes

Exercise

Schedule

5:00 _____
5:30 _____
6:00 _____
6:30 _____
7:00 _____
7:30 _____
8:00 _____
8:30 _____
9:00 _____
9:30 _____
10:00 _____
10:30 _____
11:00 _____
11:30 _____
12:00 _____
12:30 _____
1:00 _____
1:30 _____
2:00 _____
2:30 _____
3:00 _____
3:30 _____
4:00 _____
4:30 _____
5:00 _____
5:30 _____
6:00 _____
6:30 _____
7:00 _____
7:30 _____
8:00 _____
8:30 _____
9:00 _____
9:30 _____
10:00 _____
10:30 _____
11:00 _____
11:30 _____

Morning brainstorm

Big Goals

Extra Goals

Evening reflection

Day

Weight _____ BMI _____ Size _____

My mood   Drink water

☹ ☹ 😐 🙂 😃   ∪ ∪ ∪ ∪ ∪ ∪

What can I do to feel better today

_____
_____
_____
_____

Affirmation

_____
_____
_____
_____

Notes

_____
_____
_____
_____

Exercise

https://youtu.be/SvE_xFkxfJA

Schedule

Time	
5:00	
5:30	
6:00	
6:30	
7:00	
7:30	
8:00	
8:30	
9:00	
9:30	
10:00	
10:30	
11:00	
11:30	
12:00	
12:30	
1:00	
1:30	
2:00	
2:30	
3:00	
3:30	
4:00	
4:30	
5:00	
5:30	
6:00	
6:30	
7:00	
7:30	
8:00	
8:30	
9:00	
9:30	
10:00	
10:30	
11:00	
11:30	

Morning brainstorm

Big Goals

Extra Goals

Evening reflection

Day

Weight _____ BMI _____ Size _____

My mood

☹ ☹ 😐 🙂 😃

Drink water

⊌ ⊌ ⊌ ⊌ ⊌ ⊌

What can I do to feel better today

Affirmation

Notes

Exercise

Schedule

5:00 _____
5:30 _____
6:00 _____
6:30 _____
7:00 _____
7:30 _____
8:00 _____
8:30 _____
9:00 _____
9:30 _____
10:00 _____
10:30 _____
11:00 _____
11:30 _____
12:00 _____
12:30 _____
1:00 _____
1:30 _____
2:00 _____
2:30 _____
3:00 _____
3:30 _____
4:00 _____
4:30 _____
5:00 _____
5:30 _____
6:00 _____
6:30 _____
7:00 _____
7:30 _____
8:00 _____
8:30 _____
9:00 _____
9:30 _____
10:00 _____
10:30 _____
11:00 _____
11:30 _____

Morning brainstorm

Big Goals

Extra Goals

Evening reflection

Day

Weight _____ BMI _____ Size _____

My mood   Drink water

☹ ☹ 😐 🙂 😄   � � � � � �

What can I do to feel better today

Affirmation

Notes

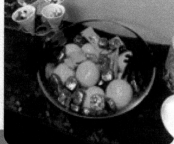

Exercise

Schedule

Time	
5:00	
5:30	
6:00	
6:30	
7:00	
7:30	
8:00	
8:30	
9:00	
9:30	
10:00	
10:30	
11:00	
11:30	
12:00	
12:30	
1:00	
1:30	
2:00	
2:30	
3:00	
3:30	
4:00	
4:30	
5:00	
5:30	
6:00	
6:30	
7:00	
7:30	
8:00	
8:30	
9:00	
9:30	
10:00	
10:30	
11:00	
11:30	

Morning brainstorm

Big Goals

Extra Goals

Evening reflection

Day

Weight _____ BMI _____ Size _____

My mood

☹ 🙁 😐 🙂 😄

Drink water

⊔ ⊔ ⊔ ⊔ ⊔ ⊔

What can I do to feel better today

Affirmation

Notes

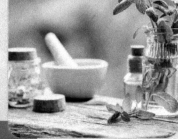

Exercise

Schedule

5:00
5:30
6:00
6:30
7:00
7:30
8:00
8:30
9:00
9:30
10:00
10:30
11:00
11:30
12:00
12:30
1:00
1:30
2:00
2:30
3:00
3:30
4:00
4:30
5:00
5:30
6:00
6:30
7:00
7:30
8:00
8:30
9:00
9:30
10:00
10:30
11:00
11:30

Morning brainstorm

Big Goals

Extra Goals

Evening reflection

Day

Weight	BMI	Size

My mood

☹ ☹ 😐 🙂 😃

Drink water

⊌ ⊌ ⊌ ⊌ ⊌ ⊌

What can I do to feel better today

Affirmation

Notes

November Challenge

If you close your Stand ring 21 times this month, you'll earn this award. Get up and get moving, Lana!

Exercise

Schedule

5:00
5:30
6:00
6:30
7:00
7:30
8:00
8:30
9:00
9:30
10:00
10:30
11:00
11:30
12:00
12:30
1:00
1:30
2:00
2:30
3:00
3:30
4:00
4:30
5:00
5:30
6:00
6:30
7:00
7:30
8:00
8:30
9:00
9:30
10:00
10:30
11:00
11:30

Morning brainstorm

Big Goals

Extra Goals

Evening reflection

Day _____

Weight _____ BMI _____ Size _____

My mood

😩 😔 😐 🙂 😄

Drink water

🥛🥛🥛🥛🥛🥛

What can I do to feel better today

_____
_____
_____
_____

Affirmation

_____
_____
_____
_____

Notes

_____
_____
_____
_____

Exercise

https://youtu.be/6OSBjfp2WRE

Schedule

Time	
5:00	
5:30	
6:00	
6:30	
7:00	
7:30	
8:00	
8:30	
9:00	
9:30	
10:00	
10:30	
11:00	
11:30	
12:00	
12:30	
1:00	
1:30	
2:00	
2:30	
3:00	
3:30	
4:00	
4:30	
5:00	
5:30	
6:00	
6:30	
7:00	
7:30	
8:00	
8:30	
9:00	
9:30	
10:00	
10:30	
11:00	
11:30	

Morning brainstorm

Big Goals

Extra Goals

Evening reflection

Day

Weight _____ BMI _____ Size _____

My mood

☹ ☹ 😐 🙂 😄

Drink water

⊔ ⊔ ⊔ ⊔ ⊔ ⊔ ⊔

What can I do to feel better today

Affirmation

Notes

Exercise

Schedule

5:00 _____
5:30 _____
6:00 _____
6:30 _____
7:00 _____
7:30 _____
8:00 _____
8:30 _____
9:00 _____
9:30 _____
10:00 _____
10:30 _____
11:00 _____
11:30 _____
12:00 _____
12:30 _____
1:00 _____
1:30 _____
2:00 _____
2:30 _____
3:00 _____
3:30 _____
4:00 _____
4:30 _____
5:00 _____
5:30 _____
6:00 _____
6:30 _____
7:00 _____
7:30 _____
8:00 _____
8:30 _____
9:00 _____
9:30 _____
10:00 _____
10:30 _____
11:00 _____
11:30 _____

Morning brainstorm

Big Goals

Extra Goals

Evening reflection

Day

Weight _____ BMI _____ Size _____

My mood

Drink water

☹ ☹ 😐 ☺ 😄

What can I do to feel better today

Affirmation

Notes

Exercise

Schedule

5:00
5:30
6:00
6:30
7:00
7:30
8:00
8:30
9:00
9:30
10:00
10:30
11:00
11:30
12:00
12:30
1:00
1:30
2:00
2:30
3:00
3:30
4:00
4:30
5:00
5:30
6:00
6:30
7:00
7:30
8:00
8:30
9:00
9:30
10:00
10:30
11:00
11:30

Morning brainstorm

Big Goals

Extra Goals

Evening reflection

Day

Weight _____   BMI _____   Size _____

My mood   Drink water

☹ ☹ 😐 🙂 😀   ⊔ ⊔ ⊔ ⊔ ⊔ ⊔

What can I do to feel better today

Affirmation

Notes

Exercise

44

Schedule

5:00	
5:30	
6:00	
6:30	
7:00	
7:30	
8:00	
8:30	
9:00	
9:30	
10:00	
10:30	
11:00	
11:30	
12:00	
12:30	
1:00	
1:30	
2:00	
2:30	
3:00	
3:30	
4:00	
4:30	
5:00	
5:30	
6:00	
6:30	
7:00	
7:30	
8:00	
8:30	
9:00	
9:30	
10:00	
10:30	
11:00	
11:30	

Morning brainstorm

Big Goals

Extra Goals

Evening reflection

Day _____

Weight _____   BMI _____   Size _____

My mood

☹ ☹ 😐 ☺ 😄

Drink water

▽ ▽ ▽ ▽ ▽ ▽

What can I do to feel better today

Affirmation

Notes

Exercise

Schedule

5:00
5:30
6:00
6:30
7:00
7:30
8:00
8:30
9:00
9:30
10:00
10:30
11:00
11:30
12:00
12:30
1:00
1:30
2:00
2:30
3:00
3:30
4:00
4:30
5:00
5:30
6:00
6:30
7:00
7:30
8:00
8:30
9:00
9:30
10:00
10:30
11:00
11:30

Morning brainstorm

Big Goals

Extra Goals

Evening reflection

Day _____

Weight _____ BMI _____ Size _____

My mood

☹ ☹ 😐 ☺ 😀

Drink water

Ḽ Ḽ Ḽ Ḽ Ḽ Ḽ

What can I do to feel better today

_____
_____
_____
_____

Affirmation

_____
_____
_____
_____

Notes

_____
_____
_____
_____

https://youtu.be/KfK3eK-kOQA

Exercise

Schedule

5:00 _____
5:30 _____
6:00 _____
6:30 _____
7:00 _____
7:30 _____
8:00 _____
8:30 _____
9:00 _____
9:30 _____
10:00 _____
10:30 _____
11:00 _____
11:30 _____
12:00 _____
12:30 _____
1:00 _____
1:30 _____
2:00 _____
2:30 _____
3:00 _____
3:30 _____
4:00 _____
4:30 _____
5:00 _____
5:30 _____
6:00 _____
6:30 _____
7:00 _____
7:30 _____
8:00 _____
8:30 _____
9:00 _____
9:30 _____
10:00 _____
10:30 _____
11:00 _____
11:30 _____

Morning brainstorm

Big Goals

Extra Goals

Evening reflection

Day

Weight _____ BMI _____ Size _____

My mood

☹ ☹ 😐 🙂 😃

Drink water

⊔ ⊔ ⊔ ⊔ ⊔ ⊔

What can I do to feel better today

Affirmation

Notes

https://youtu.be/r9jerUKJDuI

Exercise

Schedule

Time	
5:00	
5:30	
6:00	
6:30	
7:00	
7:30	
8:00	
8:30	
9:00	
9:30	
10:00	
10:30	
11:00	
11:30	
12:00	
12:30	
1:00	
1:30	
2:00	
2:30	
3:00	
3:30	
4:00	
4:30	
5:00	
5:30	
6:00	
6:30	
7:00	
7:30	
8:00	
8:30	
9:00	
9:30	
10:00	
10:30	
11:00	
11:30	

Morning brainstorm

Big Goals

Extra Goals

Evening reflection

Day

Weight   BMI   Size

My mood   Drink water

What can I do to feel better today

Affirmation

Notes

Exercise

Schedule

Time	
5:00	
5:30	
6:00	
6:30	
7:00	
7:30	
8:00	
8:30	
9:00	
9:30	
10:00	
10:30	
11:00	
11:30	
12:00	
12:30	
1:00	
1:30	
2:00	
2:30	
3:00	
3:30	
4:00	
4:30	
5:00	
5:30	
6:00	
6:30	
7:00	
7:30	
8:00	
8:30	
9:00	
9:30	
10:00	
10:30	
11:00	
11:30	

Morning brainstorm

Big Goals

Extra Goals

Evening reflection

Day

Weight _____ BMI _____ Size _____

My mood

☹ ☹ ☺ ☺ ☺

Drink water

▽ ▽ ▽ ▽ ▽ ▽

What can I do to feel better today

Affirmation

Notes

Exercise

Schedule

Time	
5:00	
5:30	
6:00	
6:30	
7:00	
7:30	
8:00	
8:30	
9:00	
9:30	
10:00	
10:30	
11:00	
11:30	
12:00	
12:30	
1:00	
1:30	
2:00	
2:30	
3:00	
3:30	
4:00	
4:30	
5:00	
5:30	
6:00	
6:30	
7:00	
7:30	
8:00	
8:30	
9:00	
9:30	
10:00	
10:30	
11:00	
11:30	

Morning brainstorm

Big Goals

Extra Goals

Evening reflection

Day

Weight _____ BMI _____ Size _____

My mood

☹ ☹ 😐 🙂 😃

Drink water

⊔ ⊔ ⊔ ⊔ ⊔ ⊔

What can I do to feel better today

Affirmation

Notes

www.higherperspectives.coml

Exercise

Schedule

5:00 ....
5:30 ....
6:00 ....
6:30 ....
7:00 ....
7:30 ....
8:00 ....
8:30 ....
9:00 ....
9:30 ....
10:00 ....
10:30 ....
11:00 ....
11:30 ....
12:00 ....
12:30 ....
1:00 ....
1:30 ....
2:00 ....
2:30 ....
3:00 ....
3:30 ....
4:00 ....
4:30 ....
5:00 ....
5:30 ....
6:00 ....
6:30 ....
7:00 ....
7:30 ....
8:00 ....
8:30 ....
9:00 ....
9:30 ....
10:00 ....
10:30 ....
11:00 ....
11:30 ....

Morning brainstorm

Big Goals

Extra Goals

Evening reflection

Day

Weight _____ BMI _____ Size _____

My mood

☹ ☹ 😐 😊 😃

Drink water

⊔ ⊔ ⊔ ⊔ ⊔ ⊔

What can I do to feel better today

Affirmation

Notes

Exercise

58

Schedule

Time	
5:00	
5:30	
6:00	
6:30	
7:00	
7:30	
8:00	
8:30	
9:00	
9:30	
10:00	
10:30	
11:00	
11:30	
12:00	
12:30	
1:00	
1:30	
2:00	
2:30	
3:00	
3:30	
4:00	
4:30	
5:00	
5:30	
6:00	
6:30	
7:00	
7:30	
8:00	
8:30	
9:00	
9:30	
10:00	
10:30	
11:00	
11:30	

Morning brainstorm

Big Goals

Extra Goals

Evening reflection

Day

Weight   BMI   Size

My mood   Drink water

What can I do to feel better today

Affirmation

Notes

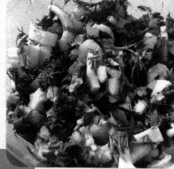

Exercise

Schedule

Time	
5:00	
5:30	
6:00	
6:30	
7:00	
7:30	
8:00	
8:30	
9:00	
9:30	
10:00	
10:30	
11:00	
11:30	
12:00	
12:30	
1:00	
1:30	
2:00	
2:30	
3:00	
3:30	
4:00	
4:30	
5:00	
5:30	
6:00	
6:30	
7:00	
7:30	
8:00	
8:30	
9:00	
9:30	
10:00	
10:30	
11:00	
11:30	

Morning brainstorm

Big Goals

Extra Goals

Evening reflection

Weight Loss Anniversary

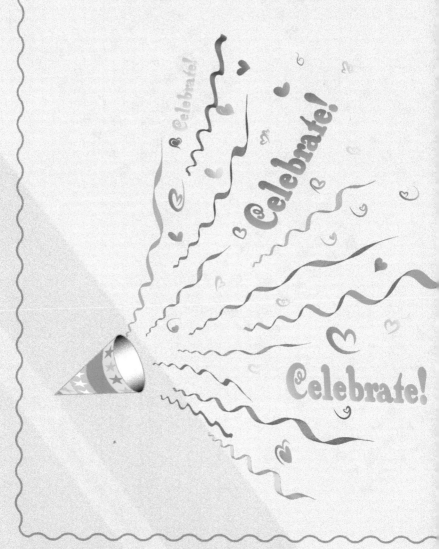

Month #1

I lost _____ pounds

I feel

Maybe I will celebrate by

_____

Day

Weight _____   BMI ____   Size _____

My mood   Drink water

☹ ☹ 😐 🙂 😃   ∀∀∀∀∀∀

What can I do to feel better today

Affirmation

Notes

Exercise

Schedule

Time	
5:00	
5:30	
6:00	
6:30	
7:00	
7:30	
8:00	
8:30	
9:00	
9:30	
10:00	
10:30	
11:00	
11:30	
12:00	
12:30	
1:00	
1:30	
2:00	
2:30	
3:00	
3:30	
4:00	
4:30	
5:00	
5:30	
6:00	
6:30	
7:00	
7:30	
8:00	
8:30	
9:00	
9:30	
10:00	
10:30	
11:00	
11:30	

Morning brainstorm

Big Goals

Extra Goals

Evening reflection

Day

Weight _____ BMI _____ Size _____

My mood

Drink water

What can I do to feel better today

Affirmation

Notes

https://youtu.be/0n3KZ7MBfYc

Exercise

Schedule

Time	
5:00	
5:30	
6:00	
6:30	
7:00	
7:30	
8:00	
8:30	
9:00	
9:30	
10:00	
10:30	
11:00	
11:30	
12:00	
12:30	
1:00	
1:30	
2:00	
2:30	
3:00	
3:30	
4:00	
4:30	
5:00	
5:30	
6:00	
6:30	
7:00	
7:30	
8:00	
8:30	
9:00	
9:30	
10:00	
10:30	
11:00	
11:30	

Morning brainstorm

Big Goals

Extra Goals

Evening reflection

Day

Weight	BMI	Size

My mood

☹ ☹ 😐 ☺ 😄

Drink water

⊔ ⊔ ⊔ ⊔ ⊔ ⊔ ⊔

What can I do to feel better today

Affirmation

Notes

Exercise

Schedule

5:00 _____
5:30 _____
6:00 _____
6:30 _____
7:00 _____
7:30 _____
8:00 _____
8:30 _____
9:00 _____
9:30 _____
10:00 _____
10:30 _____
11:00 _____
11:30 _____
12:00 _____
12:30 _____
1:00 _____
1:30 _____
2:00 _____
2:30 _____
3:00 _____
3:30 _____
4:00 _____
4:30 _____
5:00 _____
5:30 _____
6:00 _____
6:30 _____
7:00 _____
7:30 _____
8:00 _____
8:30 _____
9:00 _____
9:30 _____
10:00 _____
10:30 _____
11:00 _____
11:30 _____

Morning brainstorm

Big Goals

Extra Goals

Evening reflection

Day _____

Weight _____   BMI _____   Size _____

My mood

☹ ☹ 😐 🙂 😄

Drink water

◡ ◡ ◡ ◡ ◡ ◡

What can I do to feel better today
_____
_____
_____
_____

Affirmation
_____
_____
_____
_____

Notes
_____
_____
_____
_____

Exercise

Schedule

Time	
5:00	
5:30	
6:00	
6:30	
7:00	
7:30	
8:00	
8:30	
9:00	
9:30	
10:00	
10:30	
11:00	
11:30	
12:00	
12:30	
1:00	
1:30	
2:00	
2:30	
3:00	
3:30	
4:00	
4:30	
5:00	
5:30	
6:00	
6:30	
7:00	
7:30	
8:00	
8:30	
9:00	
9:30	
10:00	
10:30	
11:00	
11:30	

Morning brainstorm

Big Goals

Extra Goals

Evening reflection

Day

Weight _____ BMI _____ Size _____

My mood Drink water

☹ ☹ 😐 🙂 😁 ⊔ ⊔ ⊔ ⊔ ⊔ ⊔ ⊔

What can I do to feel better today

Affirmation

Notes

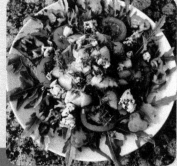

Exercise

Schedule

5:00	
5:30	
6:00	
6:30	
7:00	
7:30	
8:00	
8:30	
9:00	
9:30	
10:00	
10:30	
11:00	
11:30	
12:00	
12:30	
1:00	
1:30	
2:00	
2:30	
3:00	
3:30	
4:00	
4:30	
5:00	
5:30	
6:00	
6:30	
7:00	
7:30	
8:00	
8:30	
9:00	
9:30	
10:00	
10:30	
11:00	
11:30	

Morning brainstorm

Big Goals

Extra Goals

Evening reflection

Day _____

Weight _____   BMI _____   Size _____

My mood   Drink water

☹ ☹ 😐 🙂 😄   ⊔⊔⊔⊔⊔⊔

What can I do to feel better today
_____
_____
_____
_____

Affirmation
_____
_____
_____
_____

Notes
_____
_____
_____
_____

Exercise

Schedule

Time	
5:00	
5:30	
6:00	
6:30	
7:00	
7:30	
8:00	
8:30	
9:00	
9:30	
10:00	
10:30	
11:00	
11:30	
12:00	
12:30	
1:00	
1:30	
2:00	
2:30	
3:00	
3:30	
4:00	
4:30	
5:00	
5:30	
6:00	
6:30	
7:00	
7:30	
8:00	
8:30	
9:00	
9:30	
10:00	
10:30	
11:00	
11:30	

Morning brainstorm

Big Goals

Extra Goals

Evening reflection

Day

Weight _____ BMI _____ Size _____

My mood

😧 😞 😐 🙂 😃

Drink water

∀ ∀ ∀ ∀ ∀ ∀

What can I do to feel better today

Affirmation

Notes

https://youtu.be/gndCthN8SlY

Exercise

Schedule

Time	
5:00	
5:30	
6:00	
6:30	
7:00	
7:30	
8:00	
8:30	
9:00	
9:30	
10:00	
10:30	
11:00	
11:30	
12:00	
12:30	
1:00	
1:30	
2:00	
2:30	
3:00	
3:30	
4:00	
4:30	
5:00	
5:30	
6:00	
6:30	
7:00	
7:30	
8:00	
8:30	
9:00	
9:30	
10:00	
10:30	
11:00	
11:30	

Morning brainstorm

Big Goals

Extra Goals

Evening reflection

Day

Weight _____   BMI _____   Size _____

My mood

☹ ☹ 😐 🙂 😃

Drink water

⊔⊔⊔⊔⊔⊔

What can I do to feel better today

Affirmation

Notes

🚶	Indoor Walk	Today
	4.49MI	
🚶	Indoor Walk	Monday
	3.65MI	
🚶	Indoor Walk	Sunday
	3.59MI	
🚶	Indoor Walk	Friday
	2.52MI	
🚶	Indoor Walk	Thursday
	3.58MI	

Exercise

Schedule

Time	
5:00	
5:30	
6:00	
6:30	
7:00	
7:30	
8:00	
8:30	
9:00	
9:30	
10:00	
10:30	
11:00	
11:30	
12:00	
12:30	
1:00	
1:30	
2:00	
2:30	
3:00	
3:30	
4:00	
4:30	
5:00	
5:30	
6:00	
6:30	
7:00	
7:30	
8:00	
8:30	
9:00	
9:30	
10:00	
10:30	
11:00	
11:30	

Morning brainstorm

Big Goals

Extra Goals

Evening reflection

Day _____

Weight _____ BMI _____ Size _____

My mood

☹ ☹ 😐 ☺ 😄

Drink water

🥤 🥤 🥤 🥤 🥤 🥤

What can I do to feel better today

_____
_____
_____
_____

Affirmation

_____
_____
_____
_____

Notes

_____
_____
_____
_____

Exercise

Schedule

Time	
5:00	
5:30	
6:00	
6:30	
7:00	
7:30	
8:00	
8:30	
9:00	
9:30	
10:00	
10:30	
11:00	
11:30	
12:00	
12:30	
1:00	
1:30	
2:00	
2:30	
3:00	
3:30	
4:00	
4:30	
5:00	
5:30	
6:00	
6:30	
7:00	
7:30	
8:00	
8:30	
9:00	
9:30	
10:00	
10:30	
11:00	
11:30	

Morning brainstorm

Big Goals

Extra Goals

Evening reflection

Day _____

Weight _____   BMI _____   Size _____

My mood   Drink water

😧 😔 😐 🙂 😄   🥛 🥛 🥛 🥛 🥛 🥛

What can I do to feel better today

_____
_____
_____
_____

Affirmation

_____
_____
_____
_____

Notes

_____
_____
_____
_____

Exercise

https://youtu.be/qSkCQywDipQ

Schedule

Time	
5:00	
5:30	
6:00	
6:30	
7:00	
7:30	
8:00	
8:30	
9:00	
9:30	
10:00	
10:30	
11:00	
11:30	
12:00	
12:30	
1:00	
1:30	
2:00	
2:30	
3:00	
3:30	
4:00	
4:30	
5:00	
5:30	
6:00	
6:30	
7:00	
7:30	
8:00	
8:30	
9:00	
9:30	
10:00	
10:30	
11:00	
11:30	

Morning brainstorm

Big Goals

Extra Goals

Evening reflection

Day

Weight _____ BMI _____ Size _____

My mood

☹ ☹ 😐 ☺ 😃

Drink water

⊔ ⊔ ⊔ ⊔ ⊔ ⊔ ⊔

What can I do to feel better today

Affirmation

Notes

Exercise

Schedule

Time	
5:00	
5:30	
6:00	
6:30	
7:00	
7:30	
8:00	
8:30	
9:00	
9:30	
10:00	
10:30	
11:00	
11:30	
12:00	
12:30	
1:00	
1:30	
2:00	
2:30	
3:00	
3:30	
4:00	
4:30	
5:00	
5:30	
6:00	
6:30	
7:00	
7:30	
8:00	
8:30	
9:00	
9:30	
10:00	
10:30	
11:00	
11:30	

Morning brainstorm

Big Goals

Extra Goals

Evening reflection

Day

Weight _____ BMI _____ Size _____

My mood   Drink water

☹ ☹ 😐 🙂 😃   ⊔ ⊔ ⊔ ⊔ ⊔ ⊔

What can I do to feel better today

Affirmation

Notes

Exercise

Schedule

5:00
5:30
6:00
6:30
7:00
7:30
8:00
8:30
9:00
9:30
10:00
10:30
11:00
11:30
12:00
12:30
1:00
1:30
2:00
2:30
3:00
3:30
4:00
4:30
5:00
5:30
6:00
6:30
7:00
7:30
8:00
8:30
9:00
9:30
10:00
10:30
11:00
11:30

Morning brainstorm

Big Goals

Extra Goals

Evening reflection

Day

Weight _____   BMI _____   Size _____

My mood   Drink water

☹ ☹ ☺ ☺ ☺   ⊔⊔⊔⊔⊔⊔

What can I do to feel better today

Affirmation

Notes

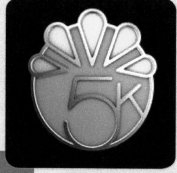

Exercise

Schedule

Time	
5:00	
5:30	
6:00	
6:30	
7:00	
7:30	
8:00	
8:30	
9:00	
9:30	
10:00	
10:30	
11:00	
11:30	
12:00	
12:30	
1:00	
1:30	
2:00	
2:30	
3:00	
3:30	
4:00	
4:30	
5:00	
5:30	
6:00	
6:30	
7:00	
7:30	
8:00	
8:30	
9:00	
9:30	
10:00	
10:30	
11:00	
11:30	

Morning brainstorm

Big Goals

Extra Goals

Evening reflection

Day

Weight _____ BMI _____ Size _____

My mood

☹ ☹ 😐 😊 😃

Drink water

⊔ ⊔ ⊔ ⊔ ⊔ ⊔

What can I do to feel better today

_____
_____
_____

Affirmation

_____
_____
_____

Notes

_____
_____
_____

Exercise

Schedule

Time	
5:00	
5:30	
6:00	
6:30	
7:00	
7:30	
8:00	
8:30	
9:00	
9:30	
10:00	
10:30	
11:00	
11:30	
12:00	
12:30	
1:00	
1:30	
2:00	
2:30	
3:00	
3:30	
4:00	
4:30	
5:00	
5:30	
6:00	
6:30	
7:00	
7:30	
8:00	
8:30	
9:00	
9:30	
10:00	
10:30	
11:00	
11:30	

Morning brainstorm

Big Goals

Extra Goals

Evening reflection

Day

Weight _____ BMI _____ Size _____

My mood   Drink water

☹ ☹ 😐 🙂 😃   ⊔ ⊔ ⊔ ⊔ ⊔ ⊔ ⊔

What can I do to feel better today

Affirmation

Notes

Exercise

Schedule

5:00
5:30
6:00
6:30
7:00
7:30
8:00
8:30
9:00
9:30
10:00
10:30
11:00
11:30
12:00
12:30
1:00
1:30
2:00
2:30
3:00
3:30
4:00
4:30
5:00
5:30
6:00
6:30
7:00
7:30
8:00
8:30
9:00
9:30
10:00
10:30
11:00
11:30

Morning brainstorm

Big Goals

Extra Goals

Evening reflection

Day

Weight _____ BMI _____ Size _____

My mood

☹ ☹ 😐 ☺ 😁

Drink water

⛢ ⛢ ⛢ ⛢ ⛢ ⛢

What can I do to feel better today

Affirmation

Notes

Exercise

Schedule

5:00	
5:30	
6:00	
6:30	
7:00	
7:30	
8:00	
8:30	
9:00	
9:30	
10:00	
10:30	
11:00	
11:30	
12:00	
12:30	
1:00	
1:30	
2:00	
2:30	
3:00	
3:30	
4:00	
4:30	
5:00	
5:30	
6:00	
6:30	
7:00	
7:30	
8:00	
8:30	
9:00	
9:30	
10:00	
10:30	
11:00	
11:30	

Morning brainstorm

Big Goals

Extra Goals

Evening reflection

Day _____

Weight _____ BMI _____ Size _____

My mood   Drink water

☹ ☹ 😐 ☺ 😃   ∪ ∪ ∪ ∪ ∪ ∪

What can I do to feel better today
_____
_____
_____

Affirmation
_____
_____
_____

Notes
_____
_____
_____

Exercise

Schedule

Time	
5:00	
5:30	
6:00	
6:30	
7:00	
7:30	
8:00	
8:30	
9:00	
9:30	
10:00	
10:30	
11:00	
11:30	
12:00	
12:30	
1:00	
1:30	
2:00	
2:30	
3:00	
3:30	
4:00	
4:30	
5:00	
5:30	
6:00	
6:30	
7:00	
7:30	
8:00	
8:30	
9:00	
9:30	
10:00	
10:30	
11:00	
11:30	

Morning brainstorm

Big Goals

Extra Goals

Evening reflection

Day

Weight _____ BMI _____ Size _____

My mood

☹ ☹ 😐 🙂 😄

Drink water

⊔ ⊔ ⊔ ⊔ ⊔ ⊔

What can I do to feel better today

_____

_____

_____

_____

Affirmation

_____

_____

_____

_____

Notes

_____

_____

_____

_____

Exercise

https://youtu.be/s5Pef_mKQ8s

Schedule

5:00 ....
5:30 ....
6:00 ....
6:30 ....
7:00 ....
7:30 ....
8:00 ....
8:30 ....
9:00 ....
9:30 ....
10:00 ....
10:30 ....
11:00 ....
11:30 ....
12:00 ....
12:30 ....
1:00 ....
1:30 ....
2:00 ....
2:30 ....
3:00 ....
3:30 ....
4:00 ....
4:30 ....
5:00 ....
5:30 ....
6:00 ....
6:30 ....
7:00 ....
7:30 ....
8:00 ....
8:30 ....
9:00 ....
9:30 ....
10:00 ....
10:30 ....
11:00 ....
11:30 ....

Morning brainstorm

Big Goals

Extra Goals

Evening reflection

Day

Weight _____ BMI _____ Size _____

My mood
☹ ☹ 😐 ☺ 😀

Drink water
⊔ ⊔ ⊔ ⊔ ⊔ ⊔

What can I do to feel better today

Affirmation

Notes

Exercise

Schedule

Time	
5:00	
5:30	
6:00	
6:30	
7:00	
7:30	
8:00	
8:30	
9:00	
9:30	
10:00	
10:30	
11:00	
11:30	
12:00	
12:30	
1:00	
1:30	
2:00	
2:30	
3:00	
3:30	
4:00	
4:30	
5:00	
5:30	
6:00	
6:30	
7:00	
7:30	
8:00	
8:30	
9:00	
9:30	
10:00	
10:30	
11:00	
11:30	

Morning brainstorm

Big Goals

Extra Goals

Evening reflection

Day

Weight _____ BMI _____ Size _____

My mood

Drink water

What can I do to feel better today

Affirmation

Notes

CTRL + ALT + DEL

Control yourself
Alter your thinking
Delete negativity

Exercise

Schedule

5:00
5:30
6:00
6:30
7:00
7:30
8:00
8:30
9:00
9:30
10:00
10:30
11:00
11:30
12:00
12:30
1:00
1:30
2:00
2:30
3:00
3:30
4:00
4:30
5:00
5:30
6:00
6:30
7:00
7:30
8:00
8:30
9:00
9:30
10:00
10:30
11:00
11:30

Morning brainstorm

Big Goals

Extra Goals

Evening reflection

Day

Weight _____   BMI _____   Size _____

My mood   Drink water

☹ ☹ 😐 ☺ 😃   ⊔⊔⊔⊔⊔⊔⊔

What can I do to feel better today

Affirmation

Notes

https://youtu.be/AVRYrrrQeds

Exercise

Schedule

Time	
5:00	
5:30	
6:00	
6:30	
7:00	
7:30	
8:00	
8:30	
9:00	
9:30	
10:00	
10:30	
11:00	
11:30	
12:00	
12:30	
1:00	
1:30	
2:00	
2:30	
3:00	
3:30	
4:00	
4:30	
5:00	
5:30	
6:00	
6:30	
7:00	
7:30	
8:00	
8:30	
9:00	
9:30	
10:00	
10:30	
11:00	
11:30	

Morning brainstorm

Big Goals

Extra Goals

Evening reflection

Day _____

Weight _____ BMI _____ Size _____

My mood

☹ ☹ 😐 ☺ 😄

Drink water

⊔ ⊔ ⊔ ⊔ ⊔ ⊔

What can I do to feel better today
_____
_____
_____
_____

Affirmation
_____
_____
_____
_____

Notes
_____
_____
_____
_____

Exercise

Schedule

5:00 _____
5:30 _____
6:00 _____
6:30 _____
7:00 _____
7:30 _____
8:00 _____
8:30 _____
9:00 _____
9:30 _____
10:00 _____
10:30 _____
11:00 _____
11:30 _____
12:00 _____
12:30 _____
1:00 _____
1:30 _____
2:00 _____
2:30 _____
3:00 _____
3:30 _____
4:00 _____
4:30 _____
5:00 _____
5:30 _____
6:00 _____
6:30 _____
7:00 _____
7:30 _____
8:00 _____
8:30 _____
9:00 _____
9:30 _____
10:00 _____
10:30 _____
11:00 _____
11:30 _____

Morning brainstorm

Big Goals

Extra Goals

Evening reflection

Day

Weight _____ BMI _____ Size _____

My mood

Drink water

😟 😦 😐 🙂 😃

What can I do to feel better today

Affirmation

Notes

Exercise

Schedule

Time	
5:00	
5:30	
6:00	
6:30	
7:00	
7:30	
8:00	
8:30	
9:00	
9:30	
10:00	
10:30	
11:00	
11:30	
12:00	
12:30	
1:00	
1:30	
2:00	
2:30	
3:00	
3:30	
4:00	
4:30	
5:00	
5:30	
6:00	
6:30	
7:00	
7:30	
8:00	
8:30	
9:00	
9:30	
10:00	
10:30	
11:00	
11:30	

Morning brainstorm

Big Goals

Extra Goals

Evening reflection

Day

Weight _____   BMI _____   Size _____

My mood   Drink water

☹ ☹ 😐 ☺ 😄   ᗡ ᗡ ᗡ ᗡ ᗡ ᗡ ᗡ

What can I do to feel better today

Affirmation

Notes

Exercise

Schedule

5:00
5:30
6:00
6:30
7:00
7:30
8:00
8:30
9:00
9:30
10:00
10:30
11:00
11:30
12:00
12:30
1:00
1:30
2:00
2:30
3:00
3:30
4:00
4:30
5:00
5:30
6:00
6:30
7:00
7:30
8:00
8:30
9:00
9:30
10:00
10:30
11:00
11:30

Morning brainstorm

Big Goals

Extra Goals

Evening reflection

Day _____

Weight _____ BMI _____ Size _____

My mood

☹ ☹ 😐 ☺ 😃

Drink water

⊔ ⊔ ⊔ ⊔ ⊔ ⊔

What can I do to feel better today

_____
_____
_____
_____

Affirmation

_____
_____
_____

Notes

_____
_____
_____

Me.

BetterMe

Exercise

Schedule

Time	
5:00	
5:30	
6:00	
6:30	
7:00	
7:30	
8:00	
8:30	
9:00	
9:30	
10:00	
10:30	
11:00	
11:30	
12:00	
12:30	
1:00	
1:30	
2:00	
2:30	
3:00	
3:30	
4:00	
4:30	
5:00	
5:30	
6:00	
6:30	
7:00	
7:30	
8:00	
8:30	
9:00	
9:30	
10:00	
10:30	
11:00	
11:30	

Morning brainstorm

Big Goals

Extra Goals

Evening reflection

Day

Weight   BMI   Size

My mood

☹ ☹ ☺ ☺ ☺

Drink water

⊔ ⊔ ⊔ ⊔ ⊔ ⊔

What can I do to feel better today

Affirmation

Notes

Exercise

https://youtu.be/cqwQosiUhTk

114

Schedule

5:00 _____
5:30 _____
6:00 _____
6:30 _____
7:00 _____
7:30 _____
8:00 _____
8:30 _____
9:00 _____
9:30 _____
10:00 _____
10:30 _____
11:00 _____
11:30 _____
12:00 _____
12:30 _____
1:00 _____
1:30 _____
2:00 _____
2:30 _____
3:00 _____
3:30 _____
4:00 _____
4:30 _____
5:00 _____
5:30 _____
6:00 _____
6:30 _____
7:00 _____
7:30 _____
8:00 _____
8:30 _____
9:00 _____
9:30 _____
10:00 _____
10:30 _____
11:00 _____
11:30 _____

Morning brainstorm

Big Goals

Extra Goals

Evening reflection

Day

Weight _____   BMI _____   Size _____

My mood   Drink water

☹ ☹ 😐 ☺ 😃   ⊎ ⊎ ⊎ ⊎ ⊎ ⊎

What can I do to feel better today

Affirmation

Notes

Exercise

Schedule

Time	
5:00	
5:30	
6:00	
6:30	
7:00	
7:30	
8:00	
8:30	
9:00	
9:30	
10:00	
10:30	
11:00	
11:30	
12:00	
12:30	
1:00	
1:30	
2:00	
2:30	
3:00	
3:30	
4:00	
4:30	
5:00	
5:30	
6:00	
6:30	
7:00	
7:30	
8:00	
8:30	
9:00	
9:30	
10:00	
10:30	
11:00	
11:30	

Morning brainstorm

Big Goals

Extra Goals

Evening reflection

Day _____

Weight _____   BMI _____   Size _____

My mood

☹ ☹ 😐 🙂 😀

Drink water

⬇⬇⬇⬇⬇⬇

What can I do to feel better today
_____
_____
_____
_____

Affirmation
_____
_____
_____
_____

Notes
_____
_____
_____
_____

Exercise

Schedule

Time	
5:00	
5:30	
6:00	
6:30	
7:00	
7:30	
8:00	
8:30	
9:00	
9:30	
10:00	
10:30	
11:00	
11:30	
12:00	
12:30	
1:00	
1:30	
2:00	
2:30	
3:00	
3:30	
4:00	
4:30	
5:00	
5:30	
6:00	
6:30	
7:00	
7:30	
8:00	
8:30	
9:00	
9:30	
10:00	
10:30	
11:00	
11:30	

Morning brainstorm

Big Goals

Extra Goals

Evening reflection

Day

Weight _____ BMI _____ Size _____

My mood

Drink water

What can I do to feel better today

Affirmation

Notes

https://youtu.be/JPFzqnpEG9A

Exercise

Schedule

Time	
5:00	
5:30	
6:00	
6:30	
7:00	
7:30	
8:00	
8:30	
9:00	
9:30	
10:00	
10:30	
11:00	
11:30	
12:00	
12:30	
1:00	
1:30	
2:00	
2:30	
3:00	
3:30	
4:00	
4:30	
5:00	
5:30	
6:00	
6:30	
7:00	
7:30	
8:00	
8:30	
9:00	
9:30	
10:00	
10:30	
11:00	
11:30	

Morning brainstorm

Big Goals

Extra Goals

Evening reflection

Day

Weight _____ BMI _____ Size _____

My mood   Drink water

☹ ☹ 😐 🙂 😄   ∪∪∪∪∪∪

What can I do to feel better today
_____
_____
_____
_____

Affirmation
_____
_____
_____
_____

Notes
_____
_____
_____

https://g.co/kgs/ywzpFK

Exercise

Schedule

5:00 _____
5:30 _____
6:00 _____
6:30 _____
7:00 _____
7:30 _____
8:00 _____
8:30 _____
9:00 _____
9:30 _____
10:00 _____
10:30 _____
11:00 _____
11:30 _____
12:00 _____
12:30 _____
1:00 _____
1:30 _____
2:00 _____
2:30 _____
3:00 _____
3:30 _____
4:00 _____
4:30 _____
5:00 _____
5:30 _____
6:00 _____
6:30 _____
7:00 _____
7:30 _____
8:00 _____
8:30 _____
9:00 _____
9:30 _____
10:00 _____
10:30 _____
11:00 _____
11:30 _____

Morning brainstorm

Big Goals

Extra Goals

Evening reflection

Weight Loss Anniversary

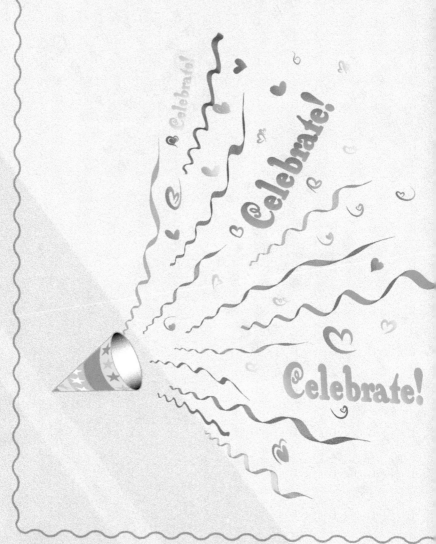

Month #2

I lost _____ pounds

I feel

Maybe I will celebrate by

_____

Day

Weight _____ BMI _____ Size _____

My mood

☹ ☹ 😐 ☺ 😃

Drink water

⊔ ⊔ ⊔ ⊔ ⊔ ⊔

What can I do to feel better today

Affirmation

Notes

Exercise

Schedule

5:00 _____
5:30 _____
6:00 _____
6:30 _____
7:00 _____
7:30 _____
8:00 _____
8:30 _____
9:00 _____
9:30 _____
10:00 _____
10:30 _____
11:00 _____
11:30 _____
12:00 _____
12:30 _____
1:00 _____
1:30 _____
2:00 _____
2:30 _____
3:00 _____
3:30 _____
4:00 _____
4:30 _____
5:00 _____
5:30 _____
6:00 _____
6:30 _____
7:00 _____
7:30 _____
8:00 _____
8:30 _____
9:00 _____
9:30 _____
10:00 _____
10:30 _____
11:00 _____
11:30 _____

Morning brainstorm

Big Goals

Extra Goals

Evening reflection

Day

Weight _____   BMI _____   Size _____

My mood   Drink water

☹ ☹ ☺ ☺ ☺   ⊔ ⊔ ⊔ ⊔ ⊔ ⊔

What can I do to feel better today
_____
_____
_____
_____

Affirmation
_____
_____
_____
_____

Notes
_____
_____
_____
_____

Exercise

Schedule

Time	
5:00	
5:30	
6:00	
6:30	
7:00	
7:30	
8:00	
8:30	
9:00	
9:30	
10:00	
10:30	
11:00	
11:30	
12:00	
12:30	
1:00	
1:30	
2:00	
2:30	
3:00	
3:30	
4:00	
4:30	
5:00	
5:30	
6:00	
6:30	
7:00	
7:30	
8:00	
8:30	
9:00	
9:30	
10:00	
10:30	
11:00	
11:30	

Morning brainstorm

Big Goals

Extra Goals

Evening reflection

Day _____

Weight _____ BMI _____ Size _____

My mood

😣 😞 😐 🙂 😀

Drink water

⊔ ⊔ ⊔ ⊔ ⊔ ⊔

What can I do to feel better today

Affirmation

Notes

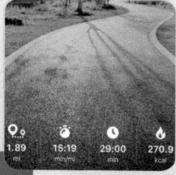

1.89
mi

15:19
min/mi

29:00
min

270.9
kcal

Exercise

Schedule

5:00 _____
5:30 _____
6:00 _____
6:30 _____
7:00 _____
7:30 _____
8:00 _____
8:30 _____
9:00 _____
9:30 _____
10:00 _____
10:30 _____
11:00 _____
11:30 _____
12:00 _____
12:30 _____
1:00 _____
1:30 _____
2:00 _____
2:30 _____
3:00 _____
3:30 _____
4:00 _____
4:30 _____
5:00 _____
5:30 _____
6:00 _____
6:30 _____
7:00 _____
7:30 _____
8:00 _____
8:30 _____
9:00 _____
9:30 _____
10:00 _____
10:30 _____
11:00 _____
11:30 _____

Morning brainstorm

Big Goals

Extra Goals

Evening reflection

Day _____

Weight _____ BMI _____ Size _____

My mood

☹ ☹ 😐 🙂 😄

Drink water

⊔ ⊔ ⊔ ⊔ ⊔ ⊔

What can I do to feel better today

Affirmation

Notes

Exercise

Schedule

Time	
5:00	
5:30	
6:00	
6:30	
7:00	
7:30	
8:00	
8:30	
9:00	
9:30	
10:00	
10:30	
11:00	
11:30	
12:00	
12:30	
1:00	
1:30	
2:00	
2:30	
3:00	
3:30	
4:00	
4:30	
5:00	
5:30	
6:00	
6:30	
7:00	
7:30	
8:00	
8:30	
9:00	
9:30	
10:00	
10:30	
11:00	
11:30	

Morning brainstorm

Big Goals

Extra Goals

Evening reflection

Day

Weight _____ BMI _____ Size _____

My mood

☹ ☹ 😐 ☺ 😄

Drink water

⊔ ⊔ ⊔ ⊔ ⊔ ⊔

What can I do to feel better today

Affirmation

Notes

Exercise

Schedule

5:00 _____
5:30 _____
6:00 _____
6:30 _____
7:00 _____
7:30 _____
8:00 _____
8:30 _____
9:00 _____
9:30 _____
10:00 _____
10:30 _____
11:00 _____
11:30 _____
12:00 _____
12:30 _____
1:00 _____
1:30 _____
2:00 _____
2:30 _____
3:00 _____
3:30 _____
4:00 _____
4:30 _____
5:00 _____
5:30 _____
6:00 _____
6:30 _____
7:00 _____
7:30 _____
8:00 _____
8:30 _____
9:00 _____
9:30 _____
10:00 _____
10:30 _____
11:00 _____
11:30 _____

Morning brainstorm

Big Goals

Extra Goals

Evening reflection

Day

Weight   BMI   Size

My mood   Drink water

☹ ☹ 😐 🙂 😄   ⊔⊔⊔⊔⊔⊔⊔

What can I do to feel better today

Affirmation

Notes

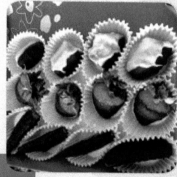

Exercise

Schedule

Time	
5:00	
5:30	
6:00	
6:30	
7:00	
7:30	
8:00	
8:30	
9:00	
9:30	
10:00	
10:30	
11:00	
11:30	
12:00	
12:30	
1:00	
1:30	
2:00	
2:30	
3:00	
3:30	
4:00	
4:30	
5:00	
5:30	
6:00	
6:30	
7:00	
7:30	
8:00	
8:30	
9:00	
9:30	
10:00	
10:30	
11:00	
11:30	

Morning brainstorm

Big Goals

Extra Goals

Evening reflection

Day _____

Weight _____   BMI _____   Size _____

My mood   Drink water
☹ ☹ 😐 🙂 😄   ⊔ ⊔ ⊔ ⊔ ⊔ ⊔

What can I do to feel better today
_____
_____
_____
_____

Affirmation
_____
_____
_____
_____

Notes
_____
_____
_____

Exercise

Schedule

Time	
5:00	
5:30	
6:00	
6:30	
7:00	
7:30	
8:00	
8:30	
9:00	
9:30	
10:00	
10:30	
11:00	
11:30	
12:00	
12:30	
1:00	
1:30	
2:00	
2:30	
3:00	
3:30	
4:00	
4:30	
5:00	
5:30	
6:00	
6:30	
7:00	
7:30	
8:00	
8:30	
9:00	
9:30	
10:00	
10:30	
11:00	
11:30	

Morning brainstorm

Big Goals

Extra Goals

Evening reflection

Day

Weight _____   BMI _____   Size _____

My mood   Drink water

☹ ☹ 😐 ☺ 😃   ⊔⊔⊔⊔⊔⊔

What can I do to feel better today

Affirmation

Notes

Exercise

Schedule

5:00 _____
5:30 _____
6:00 _____
6:30 _____
7:00 _____
7:30 _____
8:00 _____
8:30 _____
9:00 _____
9:30 _____
10:00 _____
10:30 _____
11:00 _____
11:30 _____
12:00 _____
12:30 _____
1:00 _____
1:30 _____
2:00 _____
2:30 _____
3:00 _____
3:30 _____
4:00 _____
4:30 _____
5:00 _____
5:30 _____
6:00 _____
6:30 _____
7:00 _____
7:30 _____
8:00 _____
8:30 _____
9:00 _____
9:30 _____
10:00 _____
10:30 _____
11:00 _____
11:30 _____

Morning brainstorm

Big Goals

Extra Goals

Evening reflection

Day

Weight _____   BMI _____   Size _____

My mood   Drink water

☹ ☹ 😐 ☺ 😃   ᕾ ᕾ ᕾ ᕾ ᕾ ᕾ

What can I do to feel better today

Affirmation

Notes

Exercise

Schedule

5:00 _____
5:30 _____
6:00 _____
6:30 _____
7:00 _____
7:30 _____
8:00 _____
8:30 _____
9:00 _____
9:30 _____
10:00 _____
10:30 _____
11:00 _____
11:30 _____
12:00 _____
12:30 _____
1:00 _____
1:30 _____
2:00 _____
2:30 _____
3:00 _____
3:30 _____
4:00 _____
4:30 _____
5:00 _____
5:30 _____
6:00 _____
6:30 _____
7:00 _____
7:30 _____
8:00 _____
8:30 _____
9:00 _____
9:30 _____
10:00 _____
10:30 _____
11:00 _____
11:30 _____

Morning brainstorm

Big Goals

Extra Goals

Evening reflection

Day

Weight _____ BMI _____ Size _____

My mood

☹ ☹ 😐 ☺ 😃

Drink water

▽ ▽ ▽ ▽ ▽ ▽

What can I do to feel better today

Affirmation

Notes

Exercise

Schedule

Time	
5:00	
5:30	
6:00	
6:30	
7:00	
7:30	
8:00	
8:30	
9:00	
9:30	
10:00	
10:30	
11:00	
11:30	
12:00	
12:30	
1:00	
1:30	
2:00	
2:30	
3:00	
3:30	
4:00	
4:30	
5:00	
5:30	
6:00	
6:30	
7:00	
7:30	
8:00	
8:30	
9:00	
9:30	
10:00	
10:30	
11:00	
11:30	

Morning brainstorm

Big Goals

Extra Goals

Evening reflection

Day _____

Weight _____ BMI _____ Size _____

My mood

☹ ☹ 😐 🙂 😊

Drink water

⊔ ⊔ ⊔ ⊔ ⊔ ⊔

What can I do to feel better today

_____
_____
_____
_____

Affirmation

_____
_____
_____
_____

Notes

_____
_____
_____

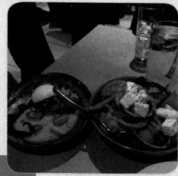

Exercise

Schedule

Time	
5:00	
5:30	
6:00	
6:30	
7:00	
7:30	
8:00	
8:30	
9:00	
9:30	
10:00	
10:30	
11:00	
11:30	
12:00	
12:30	
1:00	
1:30	
2:00	
2:30	
3:00	
3:30	
4:00	
4:30	
5:00	
5:30	
6:00	
6:30	
7:00	
7:30	
8:00	
8:30	
9:00	
9:30	
10:00	
10:30	
11:00	
11:30	

Morning brainstorm

Big Goals

Extra Goals

Evening reflection

Day

Weight _____ BMI _____ Size _____

My mood

☹ ☹ 😐 🙂 😀

Drink water

⛆ ⛆ ⛆ ⛆ ⛆ ⛆

What can I do to feel better today

Affirmation

Notes

Exercise

Schedule

Time	
5:00	
5:30	
6:00	
6:30	
7:00	
7:30	
8:00	
8:30	
9:00	
9:30	
10:00	
10:30	
11:00	
11:30	
12:00	
12:30	
1:00	
1:30	
2:00	
2:30	
3:00	
3:30	
4:00	
4:30	
5:00	
5:30	
6:00	
6:30	
7:00	
7:30	
8:00	
8:30	
9:00	
9:30	
10:00	
10:30	
11:00	
11:30	

Morning brainstorm

Big Goals

Extra Goals

Evening reflection

Day _____

Weight _____   BMI _____   Size _____

My mood

☹ ☹ 😐 🙂 😄

Drink water

⊔ ⊔ ⊔ ⊔ ⊔ ⊔

What can I do to feel better today

_____
_____
_____
_____

Affirmation

_____
_____
_____
_____

Notes

_____
_____
_____
_____

Exercise

Schedule

5:00 _____
5:30 _____
6:00 _____
6:30 _____
7:00 _____
7:30 _____
8:00 _____
8:30 _____
9:00 _____
9:30 _____
10:00 _____
10:30 _____
11:00 _____
11:30 _____
12:00 _____
12:30 _____
1:00 _____
1:30 _____
2:00 _____
2:30 _____
3:00 _____
3:30 _____
4:00 _____
4:30 _____
5:00 _____
5:30 _____
6:00 _____
6:30 _____
7:00 _____
7:30 _____
8:00 _____
8:30 _____
9:00 _____
9:30 _____
10:00 _____
10:30 _____
11:00 _____
11:30 _____

Morning brainstorm

Big Goals

Extra Goals

Evening reflection

Day

Weight _____ BMI _____ Size _____

My mood

☹ ☹ 😐 ☺ 😄

Drink water

⊔ ⊔ ⊔ ⊔ ⊔ ⊔

What can I do to feel better today

Affirmation

Notes

Exercise

Schedule

Time	
5:00	
5:30	
6:00	
6:30	
7:00	
7:30	
8:00	
8:30	
9:00	
9:30	
10:00	
10:30	
11:00	
11:30	
12:00	
12:30	
1:00	
1:30	
2:00	
2:30	
3:00	
3:30	
4:00	
4:30	
5:00	
5:30	
6:00	
6:30	
7:00	
7:30	
8:00	
8:30	
9:00	
9:30	
10:00	
10:30	
11:00	
11:30	

Morning brainstorm

Big Goals

Extra Goals

Evening reflection

Day

Weight _____ BMI _____ Size _____

My mood

☹ ☹ 😐 🙂 😄

Drink water

▙▙▙▙▙▙

What can I do to feel better today

Affirmation

Notes

Exercise

Schedule

Time	
5:00	
5:30	
6:00	
6:30	
7:00	
7:30	
8:00	
8:30	
9:00	
9:30	
10:00	
10:30	
11:00	
11:30	
12:00	
12:30	
1:00	
1:30	
2:00	
2:30	
3:00	
3:30	
4:00	
4:30	
5:00	
5:30	
6:00	
6:30	
7:00	
7:30	
8:00	
8:30	
9:00	
9:30	
10:00	
10:30	
11:00	
11:30	

Morning brainstorm

Big Goals

Extra Goals

Evening reflection

Day

Weight   BMI   Size

My mood   Drink water

☹ ☹ 😐 🙂 😄   ⊔ ⊔ ⊔ ⊔ ⊔ ⊔

What can I do to feel better today

Affirmation

Notes

Exercise

Schedule

5:00	
5:30	
6:00	
6:30	
7:00	
7:30	
8:00	
8:30	
9:00	
9:30	
10:00	
10:30	
11:00	
11:30	
12:00	
12:30	
1:00	
1:30	
2:00	
2:30	
3:00	
3:30	
4:00	
4:30	
5:00	
5:30	
6:00	
6:30	
7:00	
7:30	
8:00	
8:30	
9:00	
9:30	
10:00	
10:30	
11:00	
11:30	

Morning brainstorm

Big Goals

Extra Goals

Evening reflection

Day

Weight _____ BMI _____ Size _____

My mood

😦 😕 😐 🙂 😃

Drink water

⊔⊔⊔⊔⊔⊔⊔

What can I do to feel better today

Affirmation

Notes

Exercise

Schedule

5:00 _____
5:30 _____
6:00 _____
6:30 _____
7:00 _____
7:30 _____
8:00 _____
8:30 _____
9:00 _____
9:30 _____
10:00 _____
10:30 _____
11:00 _____
11:30 _____
12:00 _____
12:30 _____
1:00 _____
1:30 _____
2:00 _____
2:30 _____
3:00 _____
3:30 _____
4:00 _____
4:30 _____
5:00 _____
5:30 _____
6:00 _____
6:30 _____
7:00 _____
7:30 _____
8:00 _____
8:30 _____
9:00 _____
9:30 _____
10:00 _____
10:30 _____
11:00 _____
11:30 _____

Morning brainstorm

Big Goals

Extra Goals

Evening reflection

Day

Weight _____   BMI _____   Size _____

My mood   Drink water

☹ ☹ 😐 ☺ 😃   ⊔ ⊔ ⊔ ⊔ ⊔ ⊔

What can I do to feel better today

Affirmation

Notes

Exercise

Schedule

Time	
5:00	
5:30	
6:00	
6:30	
7:00	
7:30	
8:00	
8:30	
9:00	
9:30	
10:00	
10:30	
11:00	
11:30	
12:00	
12:30	
1:00	
1:30	
2:00	
2:30	
3:00	
3:30	
4:00	
4:30	
5:00	
5:30	
6:00	
6:30	
7:00	
7:30	
8:00	
8:30	
9:00	
9:30	
10:00	
10:30	
11:00	
11:30	

Morning brainstorm

Big Goals

Extra Goals

Evening reflection

Day

Weight _____ BMI _____ Size _____

My mood   Drink water

☹ ☹ 😐 ☺ 😃   ▽▽▽▽▽▽

What can I do to feel better today

Affirmation

Notes

Exercise

Schedule

Time	
5:00	
5:30	
6:00	
6:30	
7:00	
7:30	
8:00	
8:30	
9:00	
9:30	
10:00	
10:30	
11:00	
11:30	
12:00	
12:30	
1:00	
1:30	
2:00	
2:30	
3:00	
3:30	
4:00	
4:30	
5:00	
5:30	
6:00	
6:30	
7:00	
7:30	
8:00	
8:30	
9:00	
9:30	
10:00	
10:30	
11:00	
11:30	

Morning brainstorm

Big Goals

Extra Goals

Evening reflection

Day

Weight _____ BMI _____ Size _____

My mood

☹ ☹ 😐 ☺ 😄

Drink water

⊔ ⊔ ⊔ ⊔ ⊔ ⊔

What can I do to feel better today

Affirmation

Notes

Exercise

Schedule

Time	
5:00	
5:30	
6:00	
6:30	
7:00	
7:30	
8:00	
8:30	
9:00	
9:30	
10:00	
10:30	
11:00	
11:30	
12:00	
12:30	
1:00	
1:30	
2:00	
2:30	
3:00	
3:30	
4:00	
4:30	
5:00	
5:30	
6:00	
6:30	
7:00	
7:30	
8:00	
8:30	
9:00	
9:30	
10:00	
10:30	
11:00	
11:30	

Morning brainstorm

Big Goals

Extra Goals

Evening reflection

Day

Weight _____ BMI _____ Size _____

My mood

☹ ☹ 😐 ☺ 😃

Drink water

⊔ ⊔ ⊔ ⊔ ⊔ ⊔

What can I do to feel better today

Affirmation

Notes

Exercise

Schedule

5:00 _____
5:30 _____
6:00 _____
6:30 _____
7:00 _____
7:30 _____
8:00 _____
8:30 _____
9:00 _____
9:30 _____
10:00 _____
10:30 _____
11:00 _____
11:30 _____
12:00 _____
12:30 _____
1:00 _____
1:30 _____
2:00 _____
2:30 _____
3:00 _____
3:30 _____
4:00 _____
4:30 _____
5:00 _____
5:30 _____
6:00 _____
6:30 _____
7:00 _____
7:30 _____
8:00 _____
8:30 _____
9:00 _____
9:30 _____
10:00 _____
10:30 _____
11:00 _____
11:30 _____

Morning brainstorm

Big Goals

Extra Goals

Evening reflection

Day

Weight _____ BMI _____ Size _____

My mood

😖 😟 😐 😊 😄

Drink water

⊔ ⊔ ⊔ ⊔ ⊔ ⊔

What can I do to feel better today

Affirmation

Notes

Exercise

Schedule

Time	
5:00	
5:30	
6:00	
6:30	
7:00	
7:30	
8:00	
8:30	
9:00	
9:30	
10:00	
10:30	
11:00	
11:30	
12:00	
12:30	
1:00	
1:30	
2:00	
2:30	
3:00	
3:30	
4:00	
4:30	
5:00	
5:30	
6:00	
6:30	
7:00	
7:30	
8:00	
8:30	
9:00	
9:30	
10:00	
10:30	
11:00	
11:30	

Morning brainstorm

Big Goals

Extra Goals

Evening reflection

Day _____

Weight _____ BMI _____ Size _____

My mood

☹ ☹ 😐 🙂 😄

Drink water

⛆ ⛆ ⛆ ⛆ ⛆ ⛆

What can I do to feel better today

_____
_____
_____
_____

Affirmation

_____
_____
_____
_____

Notes

_____
_____
_____

Exercise

Schedule

Time	
5:00	
5:30	
6:00	
6:30	
7:00	
7:30	
8:00	
8:30	
9:00	
9:30	
10:00	
10:30	
11:00	
11:30	
12:00	
12:30	
1:00	
1:30	
2:00	
2:30	
3:00	
3:30	
4:00	
4:30	
5:00	
5:30	
6:00	
6:30	
7:00	
7:30	
8:00	
8:30	
9:00	
9:30	
10:00	
10:30	
11:00	
11:30	

Morning brainstorm

Big Goals

Extra Goals

Evening reflection

Day

Weight _____ BMI _____ Size _____

My mood

😣 😕 😐 🙂 😁

Drink water

💧💧💧💧💧💧

What can I do to feel better today

Affirmation

Notes

---

https://youtu.be/R5_TDnffZvA

Exercise

Schedule

Time	
5:00	
5:30	
6:00	
6:30	
7:00	
7:30	
8:00	
8:30	
9:00	
9:30	
10:00	
10:30	
11:00	
11:30	
12:00	
12:30	
1:00	
1:30	
2:00	
2:30	
3:00	
3:30	
4:00	
4:30	
5:00	
5:30	
6:00	
6:30	
7:00	
7:30	
8:00	
8:30	
9:00	
9:30	
10:00	
10:30	
11:00	
11:30	

Morning brainstorm

Big Goals

Extra Goals

Evening reflection

Day _____

Weight _____ BMI _____ Size _____

My mood

☹ 😟 😐 🙂 😃

Drink water

� 611 611 611 611 611

What can I do to feel better today

Affirmation

Notes

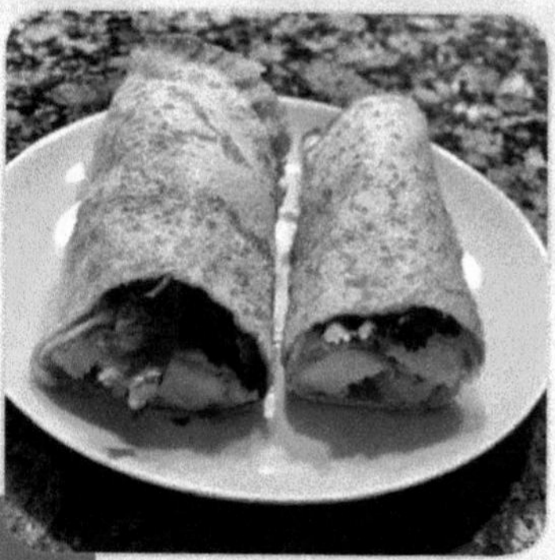

Exercise

Schedule

Time	
5:00	
5:30	
6:00	
6:30	
7:00	
7:30	
8:00	
8:30	
9:00	
9:30	
10:00	
10:30	
11:00	
11:30	
12:00	
12:30	
1:00	
1:30	
2:00	
2:30	
3:00	
3:30	
4:00	
4:30	
5:00	
5:30	
6:00	
6:30	
7:00	
7:30	
8:00	
8:30	
9:00	
9:30	
10:00	
10:30	
11:00	
11:30	

Morning brainstorm

Big Goals

Extra Goals

Evening reflection

Day _____

Weight _____ BMI _____ Size _____

My mood

☹ ☹ ☺ ☺ ☺

Drink water

ᕦᕦᕦᕦᕦᕦ

What can I do to feel better today

_____
_____
_____
_____

Affirmation

_____
_____
_____
_____

Notes

_____
_____
_____

Exercise

Schedule

Time	
5:00	
5:30	
6:00	
6:30	
7:00	
7:30	
8:00	
8:30	
9:00	
9:30	
10:00	
10:30	
11:00	
11:30	
12:00	
12:30	
1:00	
1:30	
2:00	
2:30	
3:00	
3:30	
4:00	
4:30	
5:00	
5:30	
6:00	
6:30	
7:00	
7:30	
8:00	
8:30	
9:00	
9:30	
10:00	
10:30	
11:00	
11:30	

Morning brainstorm

Big Goals

Extra Goals

Evening reflection

Day _____

Weight _____ BMI _____ Size _____

My mood

☹ ☹ 😐 ☺ 😀

Drink water

▽▽▽▽▽▽

What can I do to feel better today

_____
_____
_____
_____

Affirmation

_____
_____
_____
_____

Notes

_____
_____
_____

Exercise

Schedule

Time	
5:00	
5:30	
6:00	
6:30	
7:00	
7:30	
8:00	
8:30	
9:00	
9:30	
10:00	
10:30	
11:00	
11:30	
12:00	
12:30	
1:00	
1:30	
2:00	
2:30	
3:00	
3:30	
4:00	
4:30	
5:00	
5:30	
6:00	
6:30	
7:00	
7:30	
8:00	
8:30	
9:00	
9:30	
10:00	
10:30	
11:00	
11:30	

Morning brainstorm

Big Goals

Extra Goals

Evening reflection

Day

Weight _____ BMI _____ Size _____

My mood

😦 😔 😐 🙂 😄

Drink water

⊔ ⊔ ⊔ ⊔ ⊔ ⊔

What can I do to feel better today

Affirmation

Notes

Exercise

Schedule

Time	
5:00	
5:30	
6:00	
6:30	
7:00	
7:30	
8:00	
8:30	
9:00	
9:30	
10:00	
10:30	
11:00	
11:30	
12:00	
12:30	
1:00	
1:30	
2:00	
2:30	
3:00	
3:30	
4:00	
4:30	
5:00	
5:30	
6:00	
6:30	
7:00	
7:30	
8:00	
8:30	
9:00	
9:30	
10:00	
10:30	
11:00	
11:30	

Morning brainstorm

Big Goals

Extra Goals

Evening reflection

Day

Weight _____ BMI _____ Size _____

My mood

Drink water

$\ddot{\frown}$ $\ddot{\frown}$ $\ddot{-}$ $\ddot{\smile}$ $\ddot{\smile}$

What can I do to feel better today

Affirmation

Notes

Exercise

Schedule

Time	
5:00	
5:30	
6:00	
6:30	
7:00	
7:30	
8:00	
8:30	
9:00	
9:30	
10:00	
10:30	
11:00	
11:30	
12:00	
12:30	
1:00	
1:30	
2:00	
2:30	
3:00	
3:30	
4:00	
4:30	
5:00	
5:30	
6:00	
6:30	
7:00	
7:30	
8:00	
8:30	
9:00	
9:30	
10:00	
10:30	
11:00	
11:30	

Morning brainstorm

Big Goals

Extra Goals

Evening reflection

Day

Weight _____ BMI _____ Size _____

My mood

☹ ☹ 😐 🙂 😄

Drink water

⊔ ⊔ ⊔ ⊔ ⊔ ⊔

What can I do to feel better today

Affirmation

Notes

https://youtu.be/tjSRNhR7XOw

Exercise

Schedule

Time	
5:00	
5:30	
6:00	
6:30	
7:00	
7:30	
8:00	
8:30	
9:00	
9:30	
10:00	
10:30	
11:00	
11:30	
12:00	
12:30	
1:00	
1:30	
2:00	
2:30	
3:00	
3:30	
4:00	
4:30	
5:00	
5:30	
6:00	
6:30	
7:00	
7:30	
8:00	
8:30	
9:00	
9:30	
10:00	
10:30	
11:00	
11:30	

Morning brainstorm

Big Goals

Extra Goals

Evening reflection

Weight Loss Anniversary

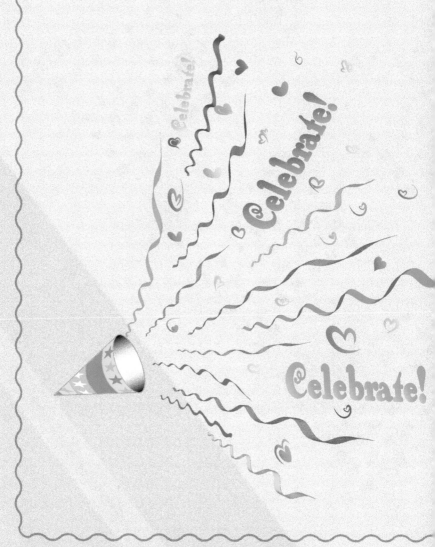

Month #3

I lost _____ pounds

I feel

Maybe I will celebrate by

_____

Testimonials & Reviews

Amazing workbook on weightloss!

Dr. Lana Moshkovich is an amazing doctor of natural medicine. I have known her for a year now and I have seen how dedicated she is to her patients and to her practice. I was so excited to hear that she had written a book about her journey to losing weight. In October 2019, Dr. Moshkovich informed me that she intended to lose weight. She took her decision and ran with it with 100% heart from the day she made this powerful decision. Every day was a step close to her goals. She made the steps easy. I saw how Dr. Moshkovich brilliantly designed a plan that would allow her to make her goals achievable.

#1 She stayed motivated every day.

#2 She stayed focused every day.

#3 She focused on her nutrition. Basically, she started really practicing what she preaches.

#4 She started using her beautiful home gym.

#5 She never made any excuses.

#6 She started a group on social media that people can join who had similar goals.

#7 She captivated her audience by each little and big goals that she achieved.

#8 She relished in her endeavors and she really celebrated every pound that she lost.

#9 She saw that her intentions far outweighed her desire to fall back to old habits.

#10 She kept at her burning desire even after she achieved her initial weightloss goals.

Dr. Moshkovich's book is simple and very easy to follow. Success leaves clues and she spells it out for the reader. There are no secrets that she keeps hidden. She really wants her readers to feel as if they CAN and WILL achieve their aspirations, and by continuing to pursue her goals, Dr. Moshkovich gives her readers and her social media followers hope that if she can do it, indeed, anyone can do it. Her goals that she lost every month were astonishing. All she had to do was stay focused and disciplined with small, deliberate and healthier choices every day.

I highly recommend Dr. Moshkovich's WEIGHT LOSS WORKBOOK

- MoveyourQi

"Fun, motivating, easy read that makes you feel like you are taking the weight loss journey with a friend."

- Karina S

"Can a person lose weight surely, steadily, and without feeling deprived? Dr. Moshkovich presents herself as Exhibit A in "Lana's Weight Loss Guide and Workbook," and answers that question with a resounding yes. Her book recounts her personal journey, and if the reader follows her daily, weekly, and monthly steps, it is absolutely possible to follow in her path to success in just three months. Her approach is holistic, since in the rest of her life, she is a Traditional Chinese Medicine doctor highly experienced with herbal remedies, nutrition, and acupuncture. Using Lana's frank confessions, motivational essays, journaling prompts, recipes, and even exercise tips that can actually be accomplished, readers have a three month program for weight loss that is destined to be successful. Reading this book is like having the personal weight loss partner you've always wanted."

- Nadiya Melnyk, DAOM, L.Ac, AMFT
  Dr. Melnyk is the founder of Wisdom of Health and author of the book Women's Health: Western and Eastern Perspective

---

"Dr. Moshkovich has designed a practical and achievable weight loss accountability program. I recommend her 90-day book to anyone that has struggled to maintain a regimented system."

- Dr. Shivali Panchal Gruer, Integrative Physician

"I have found that the best health related books are those written by authors who have personally overcome a challenge. Dr. Lana Moshkovich holds a very personal account and you can feel her passion for self-improvement throughout each day on every page. She displays lots of options, helpful suggestions, and provides a very balanced approach to the weight-loss challenge. Dr. Lana changes losing weight and improving health from one dimension to many, and encourages us to find the deeper meaning which supports our goals."

- Mariya Atrakhimovich, BSN, RN

It's well written and very inspiring and upbeat!

- J.

Success hinges on inspiration and motivation. Dr Moshkovich captures both of these elements in writing, sharing her weight loss journey with the reader in an open and honest fashion. As an experienced practitioner of Eastern medicine, Dr Moshkovich takes a holistic approach to matters of the mind and body, and understands the positive impact of sharing the weight loss journey with likeminded and positive individuals. Readers will surely feel understood and - most importantly - inspired in their own journeys.

- Irina Vigovskaya, PA-C, MMS

This planner can be followed with

Dr. Lana Weight Loss Workbook Day 1-90
Volume 1, 2, 3 or 4

Dr. Lana - YouTube Channel

https://www.youtube.com/channel/UCz16icQCVubZacMnzFnruSg

About The Author

Dr. Lana Moshkovich, DACM is a founder and director of Nirvana Naturopathics LLC.

Lana is a Licensed Acupuncturist in state of Illinois.

She holds a Doctor of Acupuncture and Chinese Medicine from Pacific College of Health and Science, San Diego, CA. She went through a 5 years of Clinical Internship in San Diego and Chicago land clinics.

She graduated as a Naturopathic Doctor and become Certified Natural Health Practitioner from Trinity College of Natural Health

Lana holds a Master of Pharmaceutical Science from Zaporizhya State Medical University, Ukraine, where she took a Hippocratic Oath.

Dr. Moshkovich and her team are focused on restoring balance to promote a healthy and happy life for all their patients.

Lana Moshkovich helps patients achieve their health and wellness goals, treating a wide range of concerns, including chronic health conditions, pain, fertility, allergies, and aging.

Certified in NAET (Nambudripad Allergy Elimination Technique)

Preferred Mei Zen Cosmetic Acupuncture Practitioner

For more information visit:

https://www.nirvananaturopathics.com

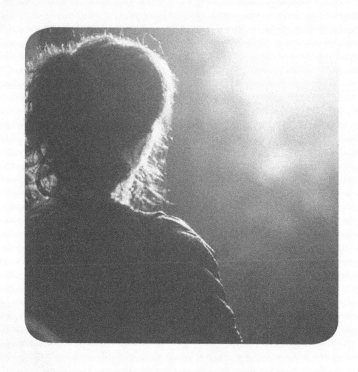

Dr. Lana Moshkovich's
90-day Wellness Planner

CPSIA information can be obtained
at www.ICGtesting.com
Printed in the USA
BVHW020242281220
596528BV00001B/1

9 781087 904702